ACID REFLUX DIET COOKBOOK

YOUR ULTIMATE GERD DIET GUIDE FOR LASTING RELIEF AND DELICIOUS WELLNESS

Ella Heartburn

INTRODUCTION

In a world loaded with culinary enjoyments and gastronomic miracles, the distress of heartburn and the unavoidable grasp of GERD can create a long-shaded area over the delight of eating. However, dread not, for inside the pages of "Dominating the Heartburn Diet," we set out on a groundbreaking excursion together—one that commitments enduring help and the rediscovery of tasty health.

Heartburn, frequently excused as a simple inconvenience, conceals a more profound truth. It is a pervasive, complex, and, once in a while, ongoing condition that can essentially influence our regular routines. Whether you've encountered periodic indigestion or grappled with the steady hand of gastroesophageal reflux infection (GERD), the excursion toward help starts here. This book is your directing light, enlightening the way to grasping heartburn and GERD in their different shades. It's an excursion into the internal functions of your stomach-related framework, an investigation of how apparently innocuous food can set off inconvenience, and a disclosure of the expansive ramifications of untreated indigestion.

However, we won't stop at information alone. "Dominating the Heartburn Diet" engages you to recover command over your well-being and prosperity. You'll figure out how to create a GERD diet plan that accommodates your one-of-a-kind necessities, stock your storeroom with the right fixings, and investigate the craft of piece control.

Through tasty GERD-accommodating recipes, you'll find that eating to mitigate side effects doesn't mean forfeiting taste. We'll dive into the world past the plate, investigating way-of-life techniques that supplement your dietary endeavors and intensify your excursion to enduring help.

This book additionally acquaints you with all-encompassing cures and normal enhancements, offering an elective way to recuperate. We'll reveal the advantages of homegrown cures, dive into the job of probiotics, and embrace the relieving properties of aloe vera and other normal cures.

Indeed, even the difficulties of eating out and traveling are tended to. You'll figure out how to explore café menus with certainty, pack beautifully for tranquil travel, and make a convenient GERD-accommodating survival kit. We accept that life ought to be enjoyed, even in a hurry. The conclusion of this book is merely the beginning of your process; it doesn't mark the end. The finishing-up section shows you the way to enduring help, offering bits of knowledge into the objective setting, progress observing, and remaining associated with a strong GERD people group.

Thus, dear peruser now is the right time to leave on your excursion to enduring alleviation and tasty health. We should divulge the mysteries of the Heartburn Diet together and reveal the delight of a daily existence unburdened by uneasiness.

Welcome to Your Excursion

Welcome to the groundbreaking excursion that is "Mastering the Acid Reflux Diet: Your Ultimate GERD Diet Guide for Lasting Relief and Delicious Wellness. As you leave on this path to a daily existence liberated from the inconvenience of indigestion, realize that you are in good company.

The excursion we embrace together is one of revelation, mending, and strengthening. An excursion perceives the intricacy of heartburn and GERD, recognizing the effect they can have on your everyday existence. Whether you've encountered periodic indigestion or confronted the tireless grasp of gastroesophageal reflux sickness (GERD), this book is your enduring buddy.

Inside these pages, we'll unwind the secrets of indigestion, offering a profound comprehension of its different structures and the cost it can take on your prosperity. Whatever the case, knowledge is only the beginning. "Dominating the Indigestion Diet" is in excess of an educational aid; it's a commonsense device to assist you with recovering command over your well-being.

You'll figure out how to create a GERD diet plan that is custom-made to your interesting necessities, load your storage room with the right fixings, and embracing the craft of part control. Also, with regards to dinners, you'll find that eating for alleviation doesn't mean forfeiting flavor. Our delightful GERD-accommodating recipes will entice your taste buds.

Be that as it may, the excursion stretches out a long way past the plate. We'll investigate way-of-life procedures that supplement your dietary endeavors, like pressure the board, standard actual work, and the significance of value rest. This book is a comprehensive aid, offering realities as well as significant advances you can take to further develop your prosperity.

We'll dive into all-encompassing cures and regular enhancements, giving an elective way to help. Homegrown cures, probiotics, and relieving aloe vera are only a couple of the devices available to you as we investigate normal ways to deal with your condition.

Indeed, even the difficulties of eating out and traveling will be tended to, guaranteeing that you can appreciate existence without being kept down by heartburn. You'll acquire the certainty to explore café menus, pack shrewdly for movement, and make a versatile GERD-accommodating survival kit.

Your process doesn't close with the last section. All things considered, it denotes the start of your way to enduring help. You'll figure out how to put forth and accomplish well-being objectives, screen your advancement, and remain associated with a steady GERD group.

Thus, think about this book as your directing light, enlightening the way to grasping heartburn, making a GERD-accommodating way of life, and embracing enduring help. Welcome to your excursion — an excursion towards heavenly health and independence from the weight of heartburn.

How This Book Can Help

As you turn the pages of "Dominating the Indigestion Diet," you'll track down something other than a book; you'll find a guide to enduring help and a better, more lively you. How about we explore this guide together?

This book is intended to give you a reasonable and extensive manual for understanding and overseeing heartburn and GERD. Our process starts with a profound plunge into these circumstances, disentangling their intricacies and revealing insight into their sweeping effect. You'll acquire bits of knowledge about their commonality and the ramifications of leaving them unmanaged.

Yet, this excursion isn't just about grasping; it's tied in with making a move. You'll figure out how to make your GERD diet plan, guaranteeing it suits your particular requirements and inclinations. We'll direct you in pursuing brilliant decisions while loading your storage room, and we'll investigate the specialty of part control to expand your solace.
Our investigation stretches out into the kitchen, where you'll find a variety of GERD-accommodating recipes that lighten side effects as well as stimulate your taste buds. Eating for help doesn't need to be dull or exhausting; it tends to be a delightful experience.

In any case, genuine help from Heartburn requires a comprehensive methodology. This book digs into way-of-life procedures that supplement your dietary endeavors. We'll examine the job of pressure, actual work, and quality snooze overseeing GERD, offering commonsense moves toward integrating these procedures into your day-to-day existence.

In our journey toward alleviation, we don't simply depend on food and our way of life. You'll likewise be acquainted with all-encompassing cures and normal enhancements, investigating elective ways to help that go beyond regular medicines.

In addition, we recognize that life is about something other than whatever you eat at home. You'll figure out how to unhesitatingly explore café menus and how to go without pressure, in any event, while managing GERD. We give pragmatic tips for feasting out and bits of knowledge about making a convenient, GERD-accommodating pack for your excursions.

At last, as you arrive at the end of this excursion, you'll not just have acquired an abundance of information and significant systems, but you'll likewise be prepared to lay out and accomplish your well-being objectives, screen your advancement, and remain associated with a strong GERD people group.

The guide to help isn't just about the objective; it's about the actual excursion. Furthermore, in this excursion, you'll learn how to recover command over your well-being and embrace enduring help and heavenly health.

Exploring the Book: Your Manual for Enduring Alleviation

As we continue to look for enduring help from indigestion, it's fundamental to have an aid that isn't just enlightening but also easy to use. This book is organized to be your confiding friend all through your excursion to understanding and overseeing heartburn and GERD.

We perceive that your time is significant, and the data you look for ought to be effectively available. To this end, the book is partitioned into unmistakable sections, each structure being the last to make a complete aid. This construction permits you to zero in on unambiguous parts of heartburn, from understanding the circumstances to making your GERD diet plan, all the way to putting forth and accomplishing your well-being objectives.

To guarantee you maximize your understanding experience, every section begins with a spellbinding snare. These snares are intended to arouse your curiosity and set up for the section's items, making your excursion through the book drawing in and educational.

In addition, all through the book, you'll find viable and significant advances as opposed to simply realities and data. We have faith in engaging you to assume command over your well-being, and that starts with furnishing you with the apparatus and information to do so. You'll track down exhortations, tips, and procedures that can be promptly carried out in your day-to-day existence.

To assist you with completely accepting the ideas and procedures introduced, we've likewise included models, individual stories, and useful delineations. These certifiable applications offer you experiences into how others have effectively dealt with their heartburn and how you can do likewise.

As you plunge into the parts, recall that your process doesn't end with the last page of this book. The finishing part gives direction on the most proficient method to commend your accomplishments, embrace another section of your life, and remain associated with a strong GERD group. Alleviation from heartburn isn't just about information; it's about the continuous help and inspiration that assist you with keeping up with your advancement and prosperity.

Thus, think of this book as a wellspring of data as well as your dependable aide on your way to enduring help and tasty health. Your process starts now, and this book is your immovable sidekick.

The Force of Assuming Command

In your mission to dominate the heartburn diet and find alleviation from the uneasiness of GERD, one thing turns out to be unmistakably clear: taking control is the way to your prosperity.

Your process is certainly not a detached one. There's no need to focus on basically figuring out indigestion; it's about effectively overseeing it. This book is your sidekick on this dynamic excursion towards enduring alleviation, where you are the driver of your fate.

By assuming command, you'll find the groundbreaking possible within your span. You have the ability to pursue decisions that decisively influence your well-being and prosperity. The choices you make, the food sources you eat, and the way of life you embrace—these components assume a critical role in overseeing heartburn.

It's an excursion where you will end up being an enabled member of your own well-being. You'll figure out how to make a GERD diet plan that lines up with your inclinations and explicit necessities—an arrangement that considers your number one flavor and dietary limitations.

Through your decisions, you can stock your storage space with the right fixings to help your dietary objectives. What's more, here you'll get familiar with the specialty of piece control, a training that guarantees your dinners are fulfilling without overburdening your stomach-related framework.

Additionally, the excursion into the kitchen will uncover how you can appreciate tasty recipes while still dealing with your condition. This book isn't tied in with denying your taste buds; it's tied in with advancing your culinary involvement in GERD-accommodating enjoyments.

Be that as it may, control stretches out past the plate. It branches into the domain of way-of-life decisions. You have some control over pressure through the different strategies that we investigate, enabling you to oversee one of the most widely recognized triggers of heartburn.

Actual work, one more part of your life under your influence, turns into an incredible asset. Exercise can improve your stomach-related well-being and, generally speaking, your prosperity. Moreover, we're here to give you counsel on how to most effectively integrate it into your daily routine.

Indeed, even something really essential can be improved to your advantage. With the right techniques and a more profound comprehension of the connection between rest and processing, you can assume command over your evening prosperity.

You'll likewise dig into comprehensive cures and normal enhancements, outfitting yourself with the information to settle on informed decisions in regard to your well-being.

This excursion shows that life isn't bound to your home or kitchen. Feasting out and voyaging are as yet a piece of your experience, and you can take control even in these circumstances. Figure out how to explore eatery menus with certainty and find the delight of movement without GERD-related pressure.

Eventually, taking control is tied in with making a feeling of dominance over your well-being, each decision in turn. This book will direct you on this excursion, giving you the apparatuses, information, and certainty to assume command and, in doing so, accomplish enduring alleviation and delectable well-being.

CHAPTER 1

UNDERSTANDING THE ACID REFLUX DIET

Heartburn, otherwise called gastroesophageal reflux disease (GERD), is a condition wherein stomach corrosive upholds enter the throat. The throat is the cylinder that associates the mouth with the stomach.

Heartburn is caused by acid reflux, which occurs when some of the stomach's acid content rushes up into the esophagus. Acid reflux on a frequent basis may be an indication of GERD.

Gastroesophageal reflux disease (GERD) happens when stomach acid runs back into the tube that connects your mouth and stomach (the esophagus). This backwash (acid reflux) can irritate the lining of your esophagus.

Many people have acid reflux on occasion. When acid reflux occurs repeatedly over time, it might lead to GERD.

The majority of people may manage their GERD symptoms with lifestyle modifications and medications. Although it is unusual, some people may require surgery to alleviate their problems.

Symptoms of Acid Reflux

GERD symptoms include the following:

A burning sensation in your chest (heartburn), which may be worse at night or while lying down.

- Food or sour liquid regurgitation (backwashing)
- Upper abdominal or chest discomfort
- Dysphagia is a problem with swallowing.

- Feeling of a lump in your throat

If you suffer acid reflux at night, you may also experience:

- A persistent cough
- Laryngitis is an inflammation of the voice chords.
- Asthma that is new or worsening

When Should You See a Doctor?

Seek immediate medical attention if you are experiencing chest discomfort, especially if you are also experiencing shortness of breath or jaw or arm pain. These could be indications of a heart attack.

Schedule a visit with your doctor if you:
- Have severe or regular GERD symptoms.
- Take over-the-counter heartburn treatments more than twice a week.

Causes of Acid Reflux

GERD is caused by frequent acid reflux or reflux of nonacidic stomach material.

When you swallow, a circular band of muscle across the bottom of your esophagus relaxes, allowing food and liquid to enter your stomach. The sphincter then closes again.

If the sphincter fails to relax or weakens, stomach acid might flow back into your esophagus. This continual acid backwash irritates your esophageal lining, leading it to become inflamed.

The following conditions can raise your risk of GERD:

- Obesity
- Hiatus hernia is a bulging of the top of the stomach above the diaphragm.

- Pregnancy
- Scleroderma and other connective tissue disorders
- Stomach emptying takes longer than usual.

The following factors can worsen acid reflux:

- Smoking
- Eating enormous amounts of food or eating late at night
- Consumption of particular foods (triggers), such as fatty or fried foods
- Consumption of certain beverages, such as alcohol or coffee
- Taking aspirin or other drugs

Complications

Chronic inflammation in your esophagus can lead to

Esophagitis (esophageal tissue inflammation) Stomach acid can cause tissue breakdown in the esophagus, resulting-inflammation) in inflammation, bleeding, and, in some cases, an open sore (ulcer). Esophagitis can cause pain and difficulty swallowing.

Esophageal stricture is a narrowing of the esophagus. Scar tissue forms in the lower esophagus as a result of stomach acid damage. The scar tissue narrows the food channel, causing swallowing difficulties.

Barrett's esophagus refers to precancerous abnormalities in the esophagus. Acid damage can induce alterations in the tissue that lines the lower esophagus. These modifications are linked to an increased risk of esophageal cancer.

What exactly is an acid reflux diet?

An acid reflux diet is a meal plan that aims to reduce acid reflux symptoms by altering one's diet and eating habits.

Benefits of the Acid Reflux Diet

The acid reflux diet has a lot of advantages, including

- **Reduced Acid Reflux Symptoms:** The acid reflux diet is intended to minimize the frequency and severity of acid reflux symptoms such as heartburn, regurgitation, and swallowing difficulties.

- **Improved Quality of Life:** Acid reflux symptoms can make it difficult to sleep, eat, and participate in activities. You can lessen your symptoms and enhance your general quality of life by following the acid reflux diet.

- **Reduced Risk of Problems:** Acid reflux can cause a variety of complications, including esophagitis (esophageal inflammation), Barrett's esophagus, and esophageal cancer. You can lower your risk of having these consequences by following the acid reflux diet.

In addition to these basic advantages, the acid reflux diet may provide additional advantages, such as:

- **Weight Loss:** Because the acid reflux diet is often low in calories and fat, it can assist you in losing weight or maintaining a healthy weight.

- **Improved Heart Health:** The acid reflux diet frequently includes fruits, vegetables, and whole grains, which can assist in enhancing heart health by lowering cholesterol levels and lowering the risk of heart disease.

- **Improved Digestive Health:** The acid reflux diet is frequently high in fiber, which can aid with digestive health and regularity.

It is critical to understand that the acid reflux diet is not a treatment for acid reflux. It can, however, be a useful technique for managing symptoms and improving quality of life. If you have acid reflux, consult your doctor about the best strategy to manage your problem.

How to Follow the Acid Reflux Diet

To follow the acid reflux diet, you should:

- Eat modest, frequent meals throughout the day. This will help lower the quantity of acid in your stomach at any given time.

- Avoid eating late at night. Eating late at night can raise the likelihood of acid reflux symptoms.

- Avoid lying down after eating. Wait at least two hours after eating before lying down. This will help prevent stomach acid from backing up into your esophagus.

- Elevate the head of your bed at night. This will help prevent stomach acid from backing up into your esophagus while you are asleep.

- Lose weight if you are overweight or obese. Excess weight can put a strain on your stomach and LES, making it more likely for acid to back up into your esophagus.

- Quit smoking. Smoking can weaken the LES and increase the amount of acid produced by the stomach.

- Manage stress. Stress might trigger acid reflux symptoms. Find healthy strategies to manage stress, such as exercise, relaxation techniques, and spending time with loved ones.

In addition to following these general suggestions, you should also avoid foods and beverages that are known to aggravate acid reflux. These include

- Fatty meals, such as fried dishes, butter, and whole milk

- Spicy foods

- Citrus fruits, such as oranges, grapefruits, and lemons

- Tomatoes

- Chocolate

- Coffee

- Tea

- Alcohol

If you are unsure whether or not a specific meal or beverage is likely to cause your acid reflux symptoms, it is advisable to err on the side of caution and avoid it.

Here are some sample meal options for the acid reflux diet:

- Breakfast: Oatmeal with berries and almonds, yogurt parfait with fruit and granola, eggs with whole-wheat bread and avocado

- Lunch: Salad with grilled chicken or fish, soup and sandwich; leftovers from dinner

- Dinner: Salmon with roasted veggies, chicken stir-fry, lentil soup

It is crucial to emphasize that the acid reflux diet is not a cure for acid reflux. However, it can be an effective strategy to manage symptoms and enhance quality of life. If you have acid reflux, it is vital to talk to your doctor about the best strategy to treat your problem.

CHAPTER 2

MEAL PLANNING AND RECIPES FOR THE ACID REFLUX DIET

Meal planning is a crucial element of following the acid reflux diet. It can assist you in ensuring that you are consuming a variety of healthful foods that are low in acid and other triggers.

Here are some recommendations for meal planning for the acid reflux diet:

1. **Start by recognizing your triggers:** What meals and beverages tend to make your acid reflux symptoms worse? Once you know what your triggers are, you may start to avoid them.

2. **Plan your meals ahead of time:** This will allow you to avoid making unhealthy choices when you are hungry.

3. **Make sure to include a variety of foods in your diet:** This will allow you to acquire the nutrition you need and avoid boredom.

4. **Eat modest, frequent meals throughout the day:** This will help to lower the quantity of acid in your stomach at any given time.

5. **Avoid foods and beverages that are known to promote acid reflux:** This includes fatty foods, spicy foods, citrus fruits, tomatoes, chocolate, coffee, tea, and alcohol.

Here are some sample meal plans for the acid reflux diet:

Breakfast

- Oatmeal with berries and nuts

- Yogurt parfait with fruit and granola

- Eggs with whole-wheat bread and avocado

- Smoothie composed of fruits, veggies, and yogurt

Lunch

- Salad with grilled chicken or fish

- Soup and sandwich

- Leftovers from supper

Dinner

- Salmon with roasted veggies

- Chicken stir-fry

- Lentil soup

- Pasta with tomato sauce and meatballs (use lean meatballs and low-acid tomato sauce)

Snacks

- Fruits and vegetables

- Nuts and seeds

- Hard-boiled eggs

- Yogurt

Here are some additional recommendations for meal planning for the acid reflux diet:

- Cook at home more often. This will give you more control over the ingredients in your food.

- Read food labels carefully. Avoid foods that include high levels of fat, sugar, and acid.

- Eat slowly and chew your food completely. This will allow your stomach to digest your food more easily.

- Avoid eating late at night. This will allow your stomach time to empty before you go to bed.

By following these guidelines, you may build a food plan that will help you control your acid reflux symptoms and enhance your overall health.

Here is a more extensive breakdown of the food plan:

Breakfast

- Oatmeal with berries and nuts: Oatmeal is a good source of fiber, which can help keep you feeling full and content. Berries and nuts are both low in acid and abundant in nutrients.

- Yogurt parfait with fruit and granola: Yogurt is a good source of protein and probiotics, which can help enhance gastrointestinal health. Fruit and granola are both low in acid and high in nutrients.

- Eggs with whole-wheat bread and avocado: Eggs are a good source of protein and healthy fats. Whole-wheat toast is a wonderful source of fiber and B vitamins. Avocado is a good source of healthy fats and fiber.

- Smoothies created with fruits, veggies, and yogurt: Smoothies are a practical way to acquire a range of nutrients in one meal. Be sure to choose fruits and vegetables that are low in acid.

Lunch

- Salad with grilled chicken or fish: Salads are an excellent method to receive a range of vitamins, minerals, and fiber. Be cautious when using a low-acid dressing. Grilled chicken or fish is a fantastic source of protein and omega-3 fatty acids.

- Soup and sandwich: Soups can be a fantastic way to receive a range of nutrients in one meal. Be cautious when choosing a low-acid soup. Sandwiches can be a healthy source of protein and fiber. Be careful to use whole-wheat bread and lean protein, such as grilled chicken or turkey.

- Leftovers from dinner: Leftovers can be a convenient and healthful route to lunch. Just be sure to avoid leftovers that are strong in acid or other triggers.

Dinner

- Salmon with roasted vegetables: Salmon is a fantastic source of protein and omega-3 fatty acids. Roasted veggies are a good source of vitamins, minerals, and fiber.

- Chicken stir-fry: Chicken stir-fries are a quick and easy way to cook a healthy supper. Be sure to use a low-acid sauce.

- Lentil soup: Lentil soup is a healthy source of protein, fiber, and iron.

- Pasta with tomato sauce and meatballs: Pasta can be a healthy source of carbohydrates and fiber. Be sure to use a low-acid tomato sauce and lean meatballs.

Snacks

- Fruits and veggies: Fruits and vegetables are a good source of vitamins, minerals, and fiber. Be sure to choose fruits and vegetables that are low in acid.

- Nuts and seeds: Nuts and seeds are a rich source of protein, healthy fats, and fiber.

- Hard-boiled eggs: Hard-boiled eggs are a wonderful source of protein and healthy fats.

- Yogurt: Yogurt is a wonderful source of protein and probiotics, which can help enhance gut health.

This is just a sample meal plan. You may need to alter it based on your specific needs and preferences. If you are unclear about what foods to eat or avoid, talk to your doctor or a qualified nutritionist.

Here are a few dishes for the acid reflux diet:

Oatmeal with Berries and Nuts

Ingredients:

- 1/2 cup rolled oats

- 1 cup water or milk

- 1/4 cup berries

- 1/4 cup chopped nuts

- 1 teaspoon honey (optional)

Instructions:

1. Combine the oats and water or milk in a saucepan.

2. Bring to a boil, then decrease the heat to low and simmer for 5 minutes, or until the oats are cooked through.

3. Stir in the berries and nuts.

4. Drizzle with honey, if preferred.

Yogurt Parfait with Fruit and Granola

Ingredients:

- 1 cup plain yogurt

- 1/2 cup fruit, such as berries, sliced bananas, or chopped apple

- 1/4 cup granola

Instructions:

1. Layer the yogurt, fruit, and granola in a jar or glass.

2. Repeat layers until the jar or glass is filled.

3. Enjoy!

Eggs with Whole-Wheat Toast and Avocado

Ingredients:

- 2 eggs

- 2 slices whole-wheat bread

- 1/4 avocado, mashed

Instructions:

1. Cook the eggs to your taste.

2. Toast the whole-wheat bread.

3. Spread the avocado on the toast.

4. Top with the eggs and enjoy!

Salad with Grilled Chicken or Fish

Ingredients:

- 2 cups mixed greens

- 1/2 cup grilled chicken or fish

- 1/4 cup chopped veggies, such as tomatoes, cucumbers, and carrots

- 2 tablespoons vinaigrette dressing

Instructions:

1. Combine the mixed greens, grilled chicken or fish, and chopped veggies in a salad bowl.

2. Drizzle with the vinaigrette dressing and toss to mix.

3. Enjoy!

Soup with Sandwich

Ingredients:

- 1 cup vegetable soup

- 1 whole-wheat sandwich with lean protein, such as grilled chicken or turkey

Instructions:

1. Heat the vegetable soup in a saucepan.

2. Assemble the whole-wheat sandwich with lean protein.

3. Enjoy the soup and sandwich together!

Leftovers from Dinner

Leftovers from dinner can be a terrific way to save time and money on meal planning. Just be sure to avoid any leftovers that are strong in acid or other triggers.

For example, if you had salmon with roasted veggies for dinner, you could pack the salmon and vegetables for lunch the next day. Or, if you had chicken stir-fry for dinner, you could pack the stir-fry for lunch the next day.

Here are some additional recommendations for cooking for the acid reflux diet:

- Use low-fat cooking methods, such as grilling, baking, or steaming.

- Avoid frying foods.

- Use herbs and spices to flavor your cuisine instead of salt.

- Avoid processed foods and sugary drinks.

By following these guidelines, you may cook delicious and healthy meals that are also excellent for your acid reflux.

Breakfast Recipes

These are some breakfast recipes that are good for the acid reflux diet:

Oatmeal with Berries and Nuts

This is a classic breakfast recipe that is both nutritious and delicious. Oatmeal is a wonderful source of fiber, which can help keep you feeling full and content. Berries and nuts are both low in acid and abundant in nutrients.

Ingredients:

- 1/2 cup rolled oats
- 1 cup water or milk
- 1/4 cup berries
- 1/4 cup chopped nuts
- 1 teaspoon honey (optional)

Instructions:

1. Combine the oats and water or milk in a saucepan.
2. Bring to a boil, then decrease heat to low and simmer for 5 minutes, or until the oats are cooked through.
3. Stir in the berries and nuts.
4. Drizzle with honey, if preferred.

Yogurt Parfait with Fruit and Granola

Yogurt is a good source of protein and probiotics, which can enhance intestinal health. Fruit and granola are both low in acid and high in nutrients.

Ingredients:

- 1 cup plain yogurt
- 1/2 cup fruit, such as berries, sliced bananas, or chopped apple
- 1/4 cup granola

Instructions:

1. Layer the yogurt, fruit, and granola in a jar or glass.
2. Repeat layers until the jar or glass is filled.
3. Enjoy!

Eggs with Whole-Wheat Toast and Avocado

Eggs are a good source of protein and healthy fats. Whole-wheat toast is a wonderful source of fiber and B vitamins. Avocado is a good source of healthy fats and fiber.

Ingredients:

- 2 eggs
- 2 slices whole-wheat bread
- 1/4 avocado, mashed

Instructions:

1. Cook the eggs to your taste.
2. Toast the whole-wheat bread.

3. Spread the avocado on the toast.
4. Top with the eggs and enjoy!

Smoothies with Fruits, Vegetables, and Yogurt

Smoothies are a practical way to receive a range of nutrients in one meal. Be sure to choose fruits and vegetables that are low in acid.

Ingredients:

- 1 cup yogurt
- 1 cup fruit, such as berries, bananas, or mango
- 1/2 cup veggies, such as spinach, kale, or cucumber
- 1/2 cup water or milk

Instructions:

1. Combine all of the ingredients in a blender and blend until smooth.
2. Enjoy!

These are just a few breakfast recipes that are good for the acid reflux diet.

Here are some additional recommendations for making breakfast for the acid reflux diet:

- Use low-fat cooking methods, such as grilling, baking, or steaming.
- Avoid frying foods.
- Use herbs and spices to flavor your cuisine instead of salt.
- Avoid processed foods and sugary drinks.
- By following these guidelines, you may produce delicious and healthy breakfast meals that are also excellent for your acid reflux.

Lunch Recipes

Lunch Recipes for the Acid Reflux Diet

Salads with Grilled Chicken or Fish

Salads are an excellent way to receive a range of vitamins, minerals, and fiber. Be cautious when using a low-acid dressing. Grilled chicken or fish is a fantastic source of protein and omega-3 fatty acids.

Ingredients:

- 2 cups mixed greens
- 1/2 cup grilled chicken or fish
- 1/4 cup chopped veggies, such as tomatoes, cucumbers, and carrots
- 2 tablespoons vinaigrette dressing

Instructions:

1. Combine the mixed greens, grilled chicken or fish, and chopped veggies in a salad bowl.
2. Drizzle with the vinaigrette dressing and toss to mix.
3. Enjoy!

Soup with Sandwich

Soups can be a fantastic way to receive a range of nutrients in one meal. Be cautious when choosing a low-acid soup. Sandwiches can be a healthy source of protein and fiber. Be careful to use whole-wheat bread and lean protein, such as grilled chicken or turkey.

Here are some examples of low-acid soups and sandwiches:

Soups:

- Chicken noodle soup

- Vegetable soup
- Lentil soup
- Tomato soup (use a low-acid tomato sauce)

Sandwiches:

- Grilled chicken sandwich on whole-wheat bread with lettuce and tomato
- Turkey sandwich on whole-wheat bread with lettuce, tomato, and avocado

Leftovers from Dinner

Leftovers from supper can be a convenient and healthy way to eat lunch. Just be sure to avoid any leftovers that are strong in acid or other triggers.

For example, if you had salmon with roasted veggies for dinner, you could pack the salmon and vegetables for lunch the next day. Or, if you had chicken stir-fry for dinner, you could pack the stir-fry for lunch the next day.

Tips for Packing Leftovers for Lunch

- Pack your leftovers in an insulated lunchbox or cooler to keep them fresh.
- If you are preparing a salad, pack the dressing separately so that the salad doesn't get soggy.
- If you are bringing soup, pack it in a thermos to keep it hot.
- If you are packing a sandwich, pack it in a reusable container to avoid using plastic wrap.

By following these guidelines, you may produce delicious and healthy lunch foods that are also excellent for acid reflux.

Dinner Recipes

Dinner Recipes for the Acid Reflux Diet

Salmon with Roasted Vegetables

Salmon is a good source of protein and omega-3 fatty acids. Roasted veggies are a good source of vitamins, minerals, and fiber.

Ingredients:

- 1 pound salmon fillet
- 1 tablespoon olive oil
- 1/2 teaspoon salt
- 1/4 teaspoon black pepper
- 1 cup broccoli florets
- 1 cup Brussels sprouts, halved
- 1/2 cup red onion, sliced

Instructions:

1. Preheat oven to 400 degrees F (200 degrees C).
2. Place the salmon fillet on a baking pan lined with parchment paper.
3. Drizzle with olive oil and season with salt and pepper.
4. Roast in the preheated oven for 12-15 minutes, or until cooked through.
5. While the salmon is roasting, toss the broccoli, Brussels sprouts, and red onion with olive oil, salt, and pepper.
6. Spread the vegetables on a baking sheet and roast in the preheated oven for 20-25 minutes, or until soft.
7. Serve the fish with the roasted veggies.

Chicken Stir-Fry

Chicken stir-fries are a quick and easy way to make a healthy supper. Be sure to use a low-acid sauce.

Ingredients:

- 1 pound boneless, skinless chicken breasts, cut into bite-sized pieces
- 1 tablespoon cornstarch
- 1 tablespoon olive oil
- 1 onion, chopped
- 2 cloves garlic, minced
- 1 red bell pepper, chopped
- 1 green bell pepper, chopped
- 1/2 cup broccoli florets
- 1/4 cup snow peas
- 1/4 cup low-acid stir-fry sauce

Instructions:

1. In a medium bowl, mix the chicken and cornstarch. Toss to coat.
2. Heat the olive oil in a large skillet or wok over medium-high heat.
3. Add the chicken and heat until browned on all sides.
4. Add the onion, garlic, bell peppers, broccoli, and snow peas to the skillet.
5. Stir-fry until the vegetables are soft.
6. Pour in the stir-fry sauce and toss to mix.
7. Cook until the sauce has thickened.
8. Serve immediately.

Lentil Soup

Lentil soup is a good source of protein, fiber, and iron.

Ingredients:

- 1 cup lentils
- 2 cups vegetable broth
- 1/2 onion, chopped
- 2 carrots, chopped
- 2 celery stalks, chopped
- 1 teaspoon garlic powder

- 1/2 teaspoon salt
- 1/4 teaspoon black pepper

Instructions:

1. Rinse the lentils in a sieve.
2. In a large pot, add the lentils, vegetable broth, onion, carrots, celery, garlic powder, salt, and pepper.
3. Bring to a boil, then decrease heat to medium and simmer for 20-25 minutes, or until the lentils are cooked.
4. Serve hot.

These are just a few dinner recipes that are good for the acid reflux diet. There are many alternative recipes available online and in cookbooks.

Here are some additional recommendations for making dinner for the acid reflux diet:

- Use low-fat cooking methods, such as grilling, baking, or steaming.
- Avoid frying foods.
- Use herbs and spices to flavor your cuisine instead of salt.
- Avoid processed foods and sugary drinks.

By following these guidelines, you may produce delicious and healthful evening foods that are also excellent for your acid reflux.

CHAPTER 3

MANAGING SPECIFIC SYMPTOMS OF ACID REFLUX

In addition to following the acid reflux diet, there are a number of things you may take to address specific symptoms of acid reflux.

Heartburn

- Elevate the head of your bed. This will assist in preventing stomach acid from backing up into your esophagus while you sleep.

- Take over-the-counter antacids or H2 blockers. Antacids neutralize stomach acid, while H2 blockers lower the quantity of acid produced by the stomach.

- Avoid lying down after eating. Wait at least two hours after eating before lying down.

- Avoid foods and beverages that trigger heartburn. Common triggers include fatty foods, spicy foods, citrus fruits, tomatoes, chocolate, coffee, tea, and alcohol.

Regurgitation

- Take over-the-counter antacids or H2 blockers. These drugs can help to minimize the amount of stomach acid that backs up into the esophagus.
- Avoid overeating. Eating too much can increase strain on the lower esophageal sphincter and make it more probable for stomach acid to back up into the esophagus.
- Avoid lying down after eating. Wait at least two hours after eating before lying down.

- Avoid meals and beverages that provoke regurgitation. Common triggers include fatty foods, spicy foods, citrus fruits, tomatoes, chocolate, coffee, tea, and alcohol.

Difficulty swallowing

- Take over-the-counter antacids or H2 blockers. These drugs can help to lessen the quantity of stomach acid that irritates the esophagus.
- Avoid consuming meals that are difficult to swallow. This may include dry foods, rough meats, and bread.
- Eat small, frequent meals. This will help to limit the amount of food in your stomach at any one moment and make it simpler to swallow.
- Avoid lying down after eating. Wait at least two hours after eating before lying down.
- Avoid foods and beverages that induce difficulty swallowing. Common triggers include fatty foods, spicy foods, citrus fruits, tomatoes, chocolate, coffee, tea, and alcohol.

If you have severe or chronic symptoms of acid reflux, it is crucial to contact a doctor. You may need to use prescription medicine to treat your symptoms.

In addition to the foregoing, there are a number of lifestyle adjustments you may adopt to help manage acid reflux symptoms. These include:

- Losing weight if you are overweight or obese. Excess weight can put a strain on the lower esophageal sphincter and make it more likely for stomach acid to back up into the esophagus.

- Quitting smoking. Smoking decreases the lower esophageal sphincter and also increases the quantity of acid produced by the stomach.

- Managing stress. Stress might trigger acid reflux symptoms. Find healthy strategies to manage stress, such as exercise, relaxation techniques, and spending time with loved ones.

By following these guidelines, you can manage the symptoms of acid reflux and enhance your quality of life.

Ways to Effectively Manage Your GERD Symptoms

GERD is one of those conditions where the abbreviation seems just as unpleasant, if not worse, than the whole medical word. Gastro-oesophageal reflux disease may be a disagreeable bodily function, to say the least, as anyone who's experienced it will know. GERD is a disorder that loosens the oesophageal sphincter, the ring of muscle around the entrance to the stomach, which then allows stomach acid to ascend up your throat, giving you an uncomfortable burning sensation. It's also preventable.

If you're hoping to find a technique to manage your GERD symptoms so you can get back to living your life, read on to discover the Rennie method for defeating GERD.

1. LOSING WEIGHT

It's never nice to be encouraged to lose weight, but if you feel that your GERD is becoming unbearable, not to mention the additional health problems that come along with obesity, then lowering your weight could be your ticket to a more comfortable existence.

Being overweight can put extra pressure on your digestive system, which can cause the valve between the stomach and the esophagus to relax, enabling stomach acid to travel upwards.

If you feel that this could apply to you, then decreasing weight would be an excellent place to start.

2. DITCH TIGHT CLOTHING

If your belt is too tight or your slim jeans are just a bit too skinny, the added pressure can drive some stomach acid into places that it shouldn't be.

A lot of GERD symptoms are avoidable, and minor modifications like these can make all the difference. If you often find yourself with GERD symptoms, then attempt to alleviate as much pressure as possible from your stomach in your day-to-day existence.

3. KEEP YOUR HEAD UP

We don't mean try to have a more positive attitude toward life, although that's never a bad thing! No, we mean physically keeping your head up.

If your symptoms are cropping up when you're attempting to sleep, then you could try elevating your bed slightly. If your head is higher than your stomach, the acid will have a harder time traveling up your esophagus and giving you that horrible burning sensation.

The upper section of your body has to be elevated, not just your head, so try raising the top legs of your bed up on some books or blocks to modify the posture of your entire body. You might also invest in a wedge cushion, which is meant to comfortably raise the entire upper half of your body.

4. GO GLUTEN-FREE

Have you considered going gluten-free? While there is no conclusive scientific consensus on the gluten-free diet, some studies have suggested that limiting the intake of foods containing high quantities of gluten, such as rye, barley, and wheat, could lead to a decrease in GERD symptoms; however, this may be due to an underlying illness.

If you've tried everything but are still dealing with GERD, then you could remove some of the more gluten-rich items from your diet and see if you notice any change.

5. WAIT BEFORE EXERCISING

If you're trying to move some pounds but find that your GERD is flaring up after exercise, then it could have something to do with your meal times.

Just like you shouldn't eat three hours before bed, you should leave time between eating and exercising. It's recommended that you wait at least two hours between a meal and indulging in physical activity, since any less means you could suffer heartburn.

These are just a few crucial actions you can take to help minimize your GERD symptoms, and while there are many more, we believe that they should give you an advantage in your quest to relieve heartburn.

Sleeping with Acid Reflux

Acid reflux, sometimes referred to as heartburn, is no stranger to most of us and is something many people struggle with every day. Four out of five people who deal with frequent heartburn are also afflicted during the night.

As we wind down and prepare our bodies for sleep, there are several aspects contributing to the quality of sleep we'll receive. However, sleeping with acid reflux can induce pain, discomfort, and ultimately weariness.

We all know the significance of getting some great shut-eye, so Rennie is setting down some facts and advice to guarantee you get quality sleep, especially with acid reflux.

BENEFITS OF SLEEP

The benefits of getting a good night's sleep are endless. Alongside the emotional joy of a nice sleep, the physical and mental benefits are what really count.

Sleep Assists

- Immune function: Helping you avoid common colds and illnesses
- Physical health: Repairing aching muscles and recovering other diseases
- Memory: Giving you the power to retain information
- Concentration: Allowing you to function and focus throughout the day
- Metabolism: Boosting your gastrointestinal system and aiding digestion
- De-stressing: Calming and calming your body and helping to limit stress

Humans require sleep to operate correctly; therefore, when acid reflux strikes, we need techniques to counteract the restless nights.

BEST SLEEPING POSITIONS FOR HEARTBURN

Left or Right?

It's preferable to sleep on your left side. Sleeping on the right has been found to relax the connecting muscles between the stomach and the esophagus. When these muscles are contracting, they aid in managing the process of acid reflux.

Front or Back?

Try to avoid sleeping on your front. This might put pressure on your stomach, which pushes acid upwards to induce heartburn. This is more likely to happen if you are overweight or obese, but you should test other positions to determine what's best for you, regardless of your weight.

Up or Down?

When lying in bed, lifting your head and shoulders a few inches helps reduce acid rising towards your chest and producing heartburn. A wedge-shaped cushion or a couple of blocks that elevate the whole upper body will perform miracles when you're attempting to sleep with acid reflux.

ACID REFLUX TOP SLEEPING TIPS

- Don't eat immediately before night - try to wait at least three hours before setting down
- Eat small meals often to help digestion - this will prevent your digestive system from being overwhelmed

- Acid reflux cures – try caffeine-free herbal teas that soothe digestion. There are various sleep-specific teas that can ease your acid reflux
- Wear comfortable clothes in bed - tight clothing can add to the pressure

in the body, inhibiting regular function and producing pain that is heightened by acid reflux

- Don't smoke. - as well as supporting poor health, smoking can make sleeping with heartburn worse by relaxing the muscles that hold acid in the stomach
- Relax and de-stress — tension leads to tight and tense muscles, which in turn impede routine bodily functions. Try meditation or time out before bed so you can release tension and snooze comfortably

Acid reflux is a frequent ailment, but trying to sleep with heartburn can be even more distressing. Try these strategies to ease your symptoms, and if the discomfort doesn't lessen, consult your doctor for further guidance.

Home Remedies to Calm Acid Reflux and Get Rid of Heartburn

There are also some established at-home therapies to help decrease acid reflux.

1. Elevate Your Upper Body While Sleeping

Acid reflux often gets worse at night, since when you lie down, it is easier for stomach acid to flow into your esophagus. You can improve nocturnal discomfort by adjusting the angle of your body during sleep.

Specifically, it is advantageous to raise your head and shoulders above your stomach and keep your esophagus tilted downward. For example, you can elevate the head of your bed or prop yourself up on a tilted pillow. "This lets gravity help clear anything that comes into the esophagus at night," adds Wolf.

A tiny 2011 study indicated that patients who elevated the head of their beds with an 8-inch block for one week reported significant improvements in their heartburn symptoms and had less disrupted sleep.

A 2016 analysis of four studies found that even for patients already taking acid reflux drugs, adding a raised sleeping posture reduced symptoms more than just taking medication alone.

To elevate your bed, you can put bed risers beneath the top two feet of your bed frame, or if this isn't possible, you can buy a sloping pillow to help angle your head and shoulders upward while sleeping.

2. Try Ingesting Deglycyrrhizinated Licorice (DGL)

Licorice is a herb that has long been used to help alleviate stomach issues. DGL is an altered kind of licorice that has had the glycyrrhizin ingredient removed, as this might elevate blood pressure.

DGL works to cure acid reflux because it helps reduce inflammation in your esophagus.

Inflammation, a reaction triggered by your immune system, can be helpful when you need to heal a wound or fight an infection, but it can also increase health problems like acid reflux for certain people. This is because your immune system generates inflammatory cells called cytokines that can damage the lining of your esophagus.

Although DGL has been proven to perform when paired with other acid reflux medications, more research is needed to discover how it works on its own.

DGL normally comes as a chewable tablet and can come in several flavors for folks who don't enjoy the taste of licorice. To use DGL for acid reflux, you should take one 400 mg tablet 20 minutes before you eat a meal or 20 minutes before going to bed if you have nighttime symptoms.

Other herbal medicines that may also help with acid reflux include:

- Ginger
- Chamomile
- Marshmallow root

3. Eat Smaller Meals

Eating heavy meals puts more strain on the sphincter that divides your esophagus from your stomach. This makes the sphincter more likely to open and allow acid to flow upward into your esophagus. Swapping up big meals for more frequent, smaller ones will help reduce your discomfort.

For example, instead of having three large meals, try spreading out those portions into five smaller meals.

4. Limit Coffee Intake

If you are a coffee drinker, cutting down or cutting out your daily cups could help minimize acid reflux. Not only is coffee already an acidic beverage, but when you drink it, your stomach is provoked into making additional stomach acid, which can become backed up and pour into your esophagus. The caffeine in coffee also causes your lower esophageal sphincter to relax, allowing stomach contents to move upward.

5. Avoid Trigger Foods

Certain foods may aggravate your acid reflux. You want to avoid foods that slow down digestion and remain in your stomach for longer, since the longer they sit, the more likely they are to increase stomach pressure and forcibly open your esophageal sphincter.

Some foods that are prone to provoking acid reflux are:

- Cheese
- Fried food
- Processed snacks like potato chips
- Fatty meats like bacon
- Chocolate

- Chili powder
- Pizza

6. Eat More Alkaline Foods

Foods that are more alkaline than acidic can balance stomach acid and help avoid reflux.

Some foods with a higher pH (indicating they are more alkaline) include:

- Cauliflower
- Fennel
- Nuts
- Bananas

7. Get More Fiber

A small 2018 study found that patients with non-erosive acid reflux illness who had a poor fiber diet lowered their incidences of acid reflux and heartburn after using psyllium fiber supplements. The extra fiber also helped enhance the esophageal sphincter's resting pressure, indicating it was less likely to relax and allow reflux through.

Also, since fiber helps you feel more full, you could be less inclined to overeat and trigger acid reflux.

However, it's not a good idea to take too much fiber or consume too many fibrous meals at once, as it might increase pressure in the gut and possibly cause reflux.

8. Sit Up After Eating

Staying upright for three hours after eating may help reduce acid reflux.

This can entail eating dinner early so you can sit up before bed or missing your after-lunch sleep.

When you're upright, gravity helps keep stomach acid in your stomach rather than in your esophagus.

9. Try sleeping on your left side

Sleeping on your left side could improve acid reflux symptoms.

A tiny 2015 study indicated that those sleeping on their left side with the upper part of their body elevated had fewer cases of acid reflux.

Meanwhile, a 2006 review listed multiple studies that suggested those who slept on their right side had worsening acid reflux.

Researchers aren't sure precisely why this is the case, but they speculate that it could be because the place where the esophagus and stomach meet is positioned above the gastric acid in the stomach when you lie on your left side

10. Take melatonin at night

A tiny 2010 study found that melatonin could relieve symptoms of gastroesophageal reflux disease (GERD) by preserving the esophagus and lowering heartburn, especially when used in conjunction with omeprazole. A person may be diagnosed with GERD if they have acid reflux often.

Additionally, a 2014 randomized controlled experiment indicated that, when taken in conjunction with omeprazole in the morning, 6 mg of melatonin taken at night relieved symptoms of functional heartburn—more so than the antidepressant nortriptyline.

A tiny 2014 study also indicated that melatonin helped maintain the esophagus's epithelial barrier, or the layer of cells that lines the esophagus, which can get destroyed with severe acid reflux.

Melatonin is presently being explored for its usage as a therapy for GERD.

You can try taking 6 mg of melatonin every night to see if it helps you. Melatonin may interfere with some medications, so if you're on any prescription medications, talk to your doctor before starting melatonin. Also, if you are pregnant, you should not take melatonin.

11. Drink Aloe Vera Juice

There is some data that indicates consuming aloe vera juice could help alleviate acid reflux.

One tiny 2015 pilot trial found that drinking 10 ml of aloe vera syrup daily helped decrease symptoms of GERD and that its benefits were comparable to the medicines ranitidine and omeprazole.

A small 2016 study focusing on male patients who developed GERD after exposure to sulfur mustard gas found that taking 40 mg of the proton-pump inhibitor pantoprazole in the morning and 5 ml of aloe vera syrup in the morning and before bed for two weeks improved the severity of GERD symptoms better than pantoprazole alone.

Proton pump inhibitors are among the strongest treatments for acid reflux. They function by reducing stomach acid levels, but long-term usage is associated with various hazards and negative effects.

The gel-like texture of aloe vera, together with its anti-inflammatory qualities, might help reduce discomfort in the gut and may help protect the organ's mucous lining.

Talk to your doctor if you're on any medication or are pregnant or breastfeeding before consuming aloe vera.

Important: Avoid the skin and inner lining of aloe vera. It contains anthraquinone, a laxative that could induce GI distress.

If you wish to try drinking aloe vera juice, search for decolorized aloe vera juice that has been processed to lower the anthraquinone concentration.

12. Try slippery elm

Slippery elm is a demulcent, meaning that it can coat and protect mucous membranes in the body. This is why it is commonly used to relieve sore throats.

In one small 2020 study, researchers gave individuals with GI issues a mixture of slippery elm, aloe vera, curcumin, guar gum, pectin, peppermint oil, and glutamine. Participants, including those with upper GI symptoms such as severe acid reflux, saw a reduction in symptoms. Researchers also pointed out that over half of the patients with upper GI symptoms were able to cease taking proton pump inhibitors at the end of the three-month study.

A tiny 2017 study had participants with stomach irritation or GERD consume a blend of slippery elm and peppermint oil. Participants reported considerable relief in symptoms and said the results were better than standard antacids.

Important: Don't take drugs within two hours of ingesting slippery elm, since it can hinder absorption.

While slippery elm eases GI issues when paired with other compounds, more research is needed to look at its benefits independent of other substances.

To use slippery elm, combine one to two tablespoons of slippery elm bark powder in a glass of water to drink after a meal or before bed. You can also purchase teas with slippery elm at various supermarkets and health food stores.

CHAPTER 4

LIFE CHANGES TO SUPPORT ACID REFLUX DIET

Heartburn, or acid reflux, is that bothersome burning sensation in your chest caused by rising gastric acid.

When you suffer from this problem on a chronic basis, it's conceivable that you have gastroesophageal reflux disease (GERD). If you smoke, you may be increasing the risk that you'll develop GERD.

GERD isn't only an uncomfortable inconvenience. It's also the major risk factor for esophageal adenocarcinoma, a cancer form. If you're looking for a reason to quit smoking and treat your GERD, keep reading to find out more.

Can smoking cause heartburn or acid reflux?

From tobacco to cannabis, there are a multitude of ways and substances that people smoke. Here's a review of some of the major categories and their possible impacts on acid reflux.

Doctors have postulated a few plausible explanations why patients who smoke report a higher incidence of heartburn or acid reflux.

- Smoking lowers lower esophageal sphincter (LES) pressure. The LES is the protective barrier that keeps acid in the stomach and out of your esophagus. When the LES pressure is lowered, the acid can more easily creep up and create heartburn.

- Smoking tobacco reduces the quantity of bicarbonate present in the saliva. Bicarbonate is an acid-neutralizing chemical.

- Smoking can increase levels of inflammation in the body. Doctors have associated increased levels of inflammation with greater risks for GERD as well as Barrett's esophagus, a condition that can lead to esophageal cancer.

There isn't a lot of data that links cannabis to GERD, or acid reflux. However, several animal studies have revealed that cannabis consumption has some good effects in relation to lowering acid reflux, including reduced gastric acid output.

Cannabis can also be used to enhance appetite and relax the stomach, but this isn't to say folks who smoke or use cannabis have no stomach problems. Some people who smoke cannabis encounter an uncommon illness called cannabinoid hyperemesis syndrome, which produces extreme vomiting.

Because vaping is somewhat new, there isn't as much information on its consequences connected to GERD.

However, there is a smaller study from Indonesia that indicated a positive association between vaping and regurgitation but a negative correlation with GERD.

While there isn't very much information about waterpipe smoking and GERD, one study found that women who smoke a waterpipe are more likely to have GERD. The study's authors didn't uncover a correlation between guys who smoked a waterpipe and greater GERD risk.

The scientists thought this was because women tend to smoke a waterpipe in greater numbers compared to men. However, scientists weren't able to pinpoint a specific explanation why women developed GERD due to smoking more than men.

There are a few rumors out on the Internet that quitting smoking can really make GERD worse instead of better, but as we've discussed, this isn't the case.

One study of 141 former smokers revealed that 43.9 percent had decreased GERD 1 year after quitting. For the control group of smokers who didn't stop, the acid reflux symptoms didn't improve with time. The researchers recommended that individuals with serious GERD cease smoking as a means to lessen their symptoms.

If the development of your GERD symptoms has coincided with quitting smoking, it likely has a separate cause that you should check with your doctor.

Can quitting smoking cause GERD?

There are a few rumors out on the Internet that quitting smoking can really make GERD worse instead of better, but as we've discussed, this isn't the case.

One study by a trusted source of 141 former smokers revealed that 43.9 percent had decreased GERD 1 year after quitting. For the control group of smokers who didn't stop, the acid reflux symptoms didn't improve with time. The researchers recommended that individuals with serious GERD cease smoking as a means to lessen their symptoms.

If the development of your GERD symptoms has coincided with quitting smoking, it likely has a separate cause that you should check with your doctor.

How to relieve heartburn

While stopping smoking should help you lessen your acid reflux symptoms, there are other treatments and home remedies that can assist as well. These include the following tips:

Avoid foods known to worsen your symptoms, such as alcohol, coffee, chocolate, fatty foods, mint, or spicy foods.
Take steps to exercise and manage your weight.
Take drugs to minimize your symptoms. These include antacids, H2 blockers

(like cimetidine or famotidine), and proton pump inhibitors (like lansoprazole and omeprazole).

Elevate your head after you eat (or elevate the head of your bed when sleeping). This inhibits acid from moving upward.

Stop eating at least 3 hours before you go to bed.

If your GERD persists, discuss it with your doctor. You may require different therapies to minimize your symptoms.

The benefits of stopping smoking for acid reflux sufferers

Quitting smoking is one of the best things you can do for your general health, and it can also have a big impact on your acid reflux symptoms.

- Smoking weakens the lower esophageal sphincter (LES). The LES is a muscle that separates the stomach from the esophagus. When the LES is weak, it can allow stomach acid to back up into the esophagus, causing heartburn and other acid reflux symptoms.
- Smoking increases gastric acid production. Smoking enhances the release of gastrin, a hormone that increases stomach acid production.
- Smoking irritates the lining of the esophagus. The esophagus is the tube that links the mouth to the stomach. Smoking can irritate the lining of the esophagus, making it more vulnerable to stomach acid.

Quitting smoking can help strengthen the LES, reduce stomach acid production, and mend the lining of the esophagus. This can lead to a dramatic improvement in acid reflux symptoms.

Tips for stopping smoking

There are many different ways to quit smoking, and the optimal approach for you will depend on your specific needs and preferences. Here are a few tips to get you started:

- Set a quit date. Choose a date in the near future and stick to it.
- Tell your friends and family that you are quitting. They can offer support and encouragement.
- Identify your triggers. What are the factors that make you want to smoke? Once you know your triggers, you may start to design techniques for avoiding them.
- Find a replacement behavior. When you have the temptation to smoke, do something else instead. This might be anything from chewing gum to going for a walk.
- Seek professional help if needed. There are many different programs and services available to help you quit smoking. Talk to your doctor or a tobacco cessation counselor about your alternatives.

Quitting smoking can be tough, but it is worth it. By stopping smoking, you can improve your general health, minimize your acid reflux symptoms, and save money.

Here are some other tips for quitting smoking:

- Avoid second-hand smoke. Second-hand smoking can trigger cravings and make it difficult to quit.
- Get rid of all of your cigarettes, lighters, and ashtrays.
- Make healthy choices. Eat a balanced diet and obtain frequent exercise.
- Find a support group. Joining a support group might help you stay motivated and connected to other individuals who are quitting smoking.

Quitting smoking is not easy, but it is achievable. Millions of individuals have quit smoking, and you can too. Remember, you are not alone. There are many people who can aid you in your quest to stop smoking.

Losing Weight

The benefits of losing weight for acid reflux sufferers Losing weight can be one of the most effective ways to manage acid reflux symptoms. Excess weight can put pressure on the stomach and lower esophageal sphincter (LES), making it more likely for stomach acid to back up into the esophagus. Losing weight can help reduce this pressure and improve acid reflux symptoms.

Tips for losing weight in a healthy way

Exercise

Dieting works best with exercise. Your GP or health advisor can help you decide how to start and how to exercise safely. You will most likely build up slowly to 30 minutes of moderate-intensity exercise on at least five days of the week. Moderate effort indicates that you are breathing somewhat more than normal, but you can still comfortably chat as you exercise. For most people, a brisk walk every day for between 30 minutes and an hour will show advantages.

A healthy diet

Weight loss should be gradual. Most specialists advocate weight loss of one to two pounds a week. Usually, doctors indicate that weight loss should be achieved by consuming roughly 600 fewer calories each day than you normally do, but this will depend on how much weight you need to drop.

A healthy diet entails swapping bad food choices, such as fast food, for healthy ones, such as fruit, vegetables, and whole grains. You should reduce your diet of fat, sugar, and alcohol and increase your intake of starchy, high-fiber meals such as wholemeal bread, brown rice, and pasta. In addition, you should consume five 80g pieces of fruit and vegetables each day. Opt for leaner cuts of meat and start steaming and boiling food instead of frying it.

When shopping, examine food labels and avoid buying products that have more than 5 grams of saturated fat per 100 grams.

Adopting a healthy, balanced diet will provide all of the calories and vital elements that the body requires, and in the long run, it will be more successful than trying to follow a fad diet.

Drug therapies

If dietary and activity adjustments have not succeeded in effectively losing weight, then doctors can prescribe medication to tackle the weight gain. The only drug currently prescribed is orlistat. This works by preventing the action of an enzyme (a protein that controls chemical events in the body) to prevent undigested fat from being absorbed into your body. Instead, the fat gets passed out with your feces (poo) - resulting in weight loss.

Where obesity is life-threatening weight loss surgery may be offered (bariatric surgery). This is a final resort. You may be offered this if you are morbidly obese with a BMI of 40+ or a BMI between 35 and 40 with an obesity-related ailment that might improve if you lose weight, such as type 2 diabetes. Surgery may involve 'gastric banding' where the stomach's size is decreased, requiring you to eat less, or gastric bypass, which modifies the way the digestive system absorbs food.

Slimming supplements

Slimming supplements such as Alli, XLS Medical Fat Binder, and Adios are approved over-the-counter supplements that are available to overweight persons aged 18 and older. Supplements should be used in conjunction with a low-calorie, low-fat diet and regular exercise. These products claim to act in various ways - some try to speed up the body's metabolic rate; others claim to reduce the body's absorption of fat.

Alternative cures and self-help

There are all kinds of therapies that people use for weight loss, but some that may prove effective include

Green tea - which contains a class of antioxidants that have been connected with improved metabolism and the capacity to affect

Fish oil - the omega-3 fatty acids in fish oil affect the way the body consumes fat. Some research suggests that instead of storing it, the body burns fat as fuel.

L-glutamine - when blood sugar levels drop, cravings tend to follow since your brain isn't getting the fuel it needs. L-glutamine quickly fuels the brain and stops the code red that makes you seek sweets and starchy meals.

Managing Stress

The link between stress and acid reflux

Stress can physically harm your body in more ways than one. Acid reflux is one of the negative affects of anxiety, and it can become a burden to your day-to-day functioning. Here are answers to some frequently asked concerns concerning stress and acid reflux that will help you comprehend their influence.

Q1. Are there specific stress-related activities that can promote acid reflux?

If you are living with anxiety or stress, it might lead to acid reflux from other lifestyle choices. Therefore, engaging in stressful activities can raise the likelihood of acid reflux. So, choose healthier choices to lessen stress levels and eliminate acid reflux problems.

Q2. Can stress management practices help decrease acid reflux symptoms?

Yes, stress management strategies like meditation, yoga, or talking to a counselor can ease your stress, thereby positively improving your whole health, including your acid reflux condition.

Q3. How can I discern between acid reflux induced by stress and other underlying factors?

If you deal with stress and worry regularly, discriminating between stress-induced acid reflux and other underlying reasons might become challenging. Therefore, you must consult your doctor or healthcare practitioner to understand your situation and get the necessary treatment.

Q4. Can continuous stress contribute to long-term consequences of acid reflux?

Chronic stress can significantly effect your overall health, including acid reflux problems. If it will effect you long-term or not, only an expert healthcare practitioner can advise you on the proper route. Therefore, get support from your doctor to deal with the situation.

Q5. Should I seek medical assistance if I feel my acid reflux is stress-related?

Yes, get medical care if you feel acid reflux has become a chronic concern. Stress-related or not, receiving the appropriate treatment at the correct time will help you lessen your acid reflux issue and eradicate it.

In conclusion, while stress may not directly cause acid reflux, strong evidence supports its involvement in worsening the condition and initiating its symptoms. Stress can alter several physiological processes, all of which can lead to acid reflux. Moreover, stress-induced behaviors such as bad eating habits and coping techniques may increase acid reflux symptoms. Therefore, controlling stress through relaxation techniques, regular exercise, good sleep, healthy food, and seeking assistance can be helpful in lowering the influence of stress on acid reflux, encouraging improved gastrointestinal health, and boosting overall well-being.

Tips for handling stress

There are a lot of things you can do to manage stress and lower your risk of acid reflux symptoms. Here are a few tips:

- Exercise regularly. Exercise is a terrific strategy to alleviate stress and enhance your overall health. Aim for at least 30 minutes of moderate-intensity exercise most days of the week.
- Get adequate sleep. When you are well-rested, you are better able to cope with stress. Aim for 7-8 hours of sleep per night.
- Eat a nutritious diet. Eating a balanced diet can help boost your mood and reduce stress levels. Avoid processed foods, fizzy drinks, and harmful fats. Focus on eating plenty of fruits, veggies, and whole grains.
- Practice relaxing techniques. There are a lot of relaxation practices that can help relieve stress, such as deep breathing, meditation, and yoga. Find a relaxing method that works for you and practice it often.

If you are struggling to handle stress on your own, go to your doctor or a therapist. They can help you build a stress management plan that is perfect for you.

Here are some other strategies for handling stress:

- Identify your stressors. What are the things that give you stress? Once you know your stressors, you may start to establish ways of coping with them.
- Take breaks. If you are feeling overwhelmed, take a few minutes to relax and clear your head. Go for a walk, listen to music, or read a book.
- Say no. It's alright to say no to requests if you don't have the time or energy to take them on.
- Ask for aid. Don't be reluctant to seek support from friends, family, or professionals.

Managing stress is vital for your entire health and well-being. By following these strategies, you can minimize stress and improve your acid reflux symptoms.

Avoiding Eating Late at Night

The benefits of avoiding eating late at night for acid reflux sufferers

Eating late at night can raise your chance of acid reflux symptoms. When you eat late at night, your stomach has less time to empty before you go to bed. This can give stomach acid more time to back up into the esophagus, causing heartburn and other acid reflux symptoms.

In addition, when you lie down after eating, gravity can make it easier for stomach acid to back up into the esophagus.

Avoiding eating late at night can help lower your risk of acid reflux symptoms and enhance your sleep quality.

Tips for avoiding eating late at night

Here are a few ideas for avoiding eating late at night:

- Eat dinner early in the evening. Aim to finish dinner at least 3 hours before you go to bed.
- Avoid late-night snacking. If you feel hungry before bed, have a light snack, such as a piece of fruit or yogurt.
- Don't go to bed hungry. If you go to bed hungry, you are more likely to wake up in the middle of the night and eat.
- Identify your triggers. What are the factors that make you want to eat late at night? Once you know your triggers, you may start to design techniques for avoiding them.

Here are some other strategies for avoiding eating late at night:

- Brush your teeth after meals. This will help to convey to your brain that you are finished eating for the day.
- Avoid watching TV or using electronic devices in bed. The blue light emitted from these devices can interfere with sleep and make it more likely that you will crave food late at night.
- Create a calm nighttime routine. This could include taking a warm bath, reading a book, or listening to calming music.

- Make sure your bedroom is dark, quiet, and cool. This will help establish an environment that is suitable to sleeping

.

Avoiding eating late at night can be tough, but it is worth it for your general health and well-being. By following these tips, you can lower your risk of acid reflux symptoms and enhance your sleep quality.

Elevating the Head of Your Bed at Night

The benefits of elevating the head of your bed at night for acid reflux patients

Elevating the head of your bed at night can help lower your chance of acid reflux symptoms. When you elevate the head of your bed, gravity helps to prevent stomach acid from backing up into the esophagus.

Elevating the head of your bed can also help improve your sleep quality. When you have acid reflux symptoms, it might be difficult to get a decent night's sleep. Elevating the head of your bed can help minimize your acid reflux symptoms and make it easier to fall asleep and remain asleep.

Tips for elevating the head of your bed at night

There are a lot of techniques to elevate the head of your bed at night. Here are a few tips:

- Use a wedge pillow. A wedge pillow is a triangular-shaped pillow that can be positioned under your head and shoulders to raise your upper torso.
- Place a stack of cushions under your head and shoulders. If you don't have a wedge pillow, you can use a stack of pillows to raise your upper body.
- Raise the head of your bed frame. Some bed frames have movable headboards that allow you to raise the head of your bed.
- Use a recliner. If you have a recliner, you can recline at a comfortable angle to raise your upper body.

When raising the head of your bed, it is vital to start with a small angle and progressively increase the angle until you find a comfortable posture. You may also want to place a pillow between your knees to help support your spine.

Here are some extra tips for elevating the head of your bed at night:

- Use a firm pillow. A firm pillow will help to keep your neck and spine in alignment.
- Avoid using too many pillows. Too many pillows might put your neck and spine in an awkward position.
- Listen to your body. If you encounter any pain or discomfort, discontinue lifting the head of your bed.

Elevating the head of your bed at night is a simple and effective strategy to lower your risk of acid reflux symptoms and enhance your sleep quality. By following these guidelines, you can find a comfortable and safe way to elevate the head of your bed at night.

CHAPTER 5

COMMON HEARTBURN MYTHS AND FACTS

There is a lot of inaccurate information out there regarding heartburn, what it could imply, and how to cure it. This will help you identify heartbreaking truths from misconceptions!

Myth #1: Heartburn is a Sign of a Heart Attack

Fact: False. Heartburn is a sign of acid reflux, a condition in which acidic fluid from the stomach backs up into the esophagus, or swallowing tube. It is not caused by a heart issue. The discomfort of heartburn is often linked with a burning sensation exactly beneath the breastbone, causing many people to immediately think it is related to the heart, when it is not. The discomfort is generally accompanied by burping, signs of bloating, or gas. Sometimes, an acid taste occurs in the mouth. Heartburn symptoms often develop worse after eating a heavy meal, using tobacco, or consuming alcohol or caffeine, and tend to improve after taking antacids. Keep in mind that while heartburn can produce chest pain around your heart, this ailment is not heart linked. The symptoms of heartburn and heart attack are extremely distinct but can feel similar. It is crucial to know when to seek medical treatment.

Myth #2: Chewing Gum Can Ease My Heartburn
Fact: True. When you chew gum, your mouth creates saliva, which acts as a natural barrier to acid. It may help ease the burning feeling you may experience when you acquire heartburn. Discover more about the numerous strategies to help minimize your heartburn symptoms.

Myth #3: Milk or Cream Calms Heartburn Symptoms

Fact: False. Based on the newest scientific data, doctors do not recommend drinking milk or cream to relieve heartburn. It has been found that milk momentarily reduces heartburn symptoms only to later boost acid production in the stomach, which produces additional heartburn.

Myth #4: Heartburn is no big deal. It is Just a Minor, Trivial Complaint

Fact: False. Heartburn is prevalent, but it is not trivial! In reality, recurrent heartburn can adversely influence your quality of life, productivity, and daily activities. Besides, persistent heartburn that occurs more than twice a week could be an indication of a more serious condition called GERD, which, if left untreated, can contribute to a wide variety of disorders such as ulcers of the esophagus, asthma, and chronic cough. These risks may be avoided with adequate supervision from a physician. Remember, people with heartburn do not need to suffer in silence. Changes in food and lifestyle, as well as a fast-growing selection of over-the-counter (OTC) and prescription drugs, can provide relief for most heartburn sufferers. Talk to your doctor if you think you may be experiencing any of these issues and/or if you want to turn to OTC heartburn treatment choices.

Myth #5: Heartburn is My Fault

Fact: False. Heartburn is a medical ailment with actual biological reasons, and those who suffer from heartburn should not compound their misery with shame and guilt. While it is true that certain lifestyle choices and the foods and beverages you consume and drink might aggravate your heartburn symptoms, many people make significant lifestyle adjustments to battle heartburn yet still have heartburn symptoms. Once again, heartburn is not your fault, and there are various ways you can manage the discomfort of heartburn through lifestyle modifications and OTC drugs.

Myth #6: I Will Always Have to Live with Heartburn and It Will Never Go Away

Fact: False. Heartburn affects roughly 20 percent of the population in the U.S., and experiencing heartburn once in a while is common, but suffering from nocturnal heartburn or frequent heartburn on two or more days per week can have a huge impact on your life. While there may be no proven cure for heartburn, several OTC medications can truly stop heartburn and provide long-lasting symptom relief. H2-blockers like Pepcid® can help lower acid for up to 12 hours. Proton pump inhibitors (Eg. Omeprazole, available at Curist here; Esomeprazole, available at Curist here) more effectively inhibit acid production and offer 24-hour symptom relief from heartburn with one daily pill, so you can go about your daily life without constantly worrying about your symptoms.

Myth #7: If I Take a Drug to Suppress Acid Production, I Won't Be Able to Digest My Food Fact: False. Our bodies produce stomach acid to help break down proteins, carbs, and fat from the food in the stomach and to destroy microorganisms. Even OTC proton pump inhibitors (e.g., Omeprazole, available at Curist here; Esomeprazole, available at Curist here), which work directly on active acid pumps in the stomach to considerably restrict acid production, allow enough acid to be created so that normal food digestion occurs.

CHAPTER 6

LONG-TERM SUCCESS ON THE ACID RELUX DIET

Following the acid reflux diet for the long run can be tough, but it is worth it to manage your symptoms and enhance your general health. Here are some strategies for keeping motivated, handling setbacks, and getting support:

Steps to Living a Happier Life with GERD

Change your eating routine.

Eat smaller portions. For example, six small meals may be good as opposed to three larger ones. Keeping your stomach from being overly full minimizes gastric pressure.

Similarly, eating slower helps by putting less food in your stomach at one time.

It is also vital to know what meals may provoke reflux. Some of the things more likely to trigger reflux are tea, carbonated beverages, coffee, alcohol, mint, spicy foods, fatty foods, tomatoes, garlic, onions, and chocolate. If you routinely consume these items, consider eliminating them from your diet and gently reintroducing them one by one to establish which foods worsen your GERD symptoms.

Lose weight if you need to

Eating slowly may also help you lose weight,, if this is something you need to do. Excessive weight causes the muscular tissue that supports the lower esophageal sphincter to expand. This subsequently lessens the pressure, which maintains the sphincter closed, leading to reflux and heartburn.

Limit activity after eating

Avoiding intense workouts for a couple hours after eating may keep symptoms at bay. Any exercises that involve bending over should especially be avoided, as it sends acid into the esophagus.

Stop smoking

Nicotine can relax the lower esophageal sphincter, aggravating heartburn.

Change your sleep habits

Staying awake for 2-3 hours after eating can help, as gravity and food digestion work together to reduce symptoms. Sleeping with your head and shoulders elevated- either by pillows or in a chair- also helps alleviate pressure and keep stomach contents where they belong.

Review your medications.

Some drugs might relax the sphincter, while others can irritate the esophagus. Over the counter antacids can considerably alleviate heartburn but should not be used consistently. Consult with your physician to explore which prescriptions you may need to take or adjust to minimize your symptoms.

Check your clothes

Tight-fitting garments around the abdomen should be avoided. This includes tight belts, jeans, and slender undergarments.

Relax

Learning relaxation skills may help alleviate tension. Although stress has not been related to heartburn, it can lead to heartburn causing behaviors.

Tips for remaining motivated

- Set reasonable goals. Don't try to alter everything at once. Start by making tiny modifications to your food and lifestyle. You can progressively add more adjustments as you get more comfortable.
- Focus on the benefits. Remind yourself of the reasons why you are following the acid reflux diet. Think about how treating your symptoms will improve your quality of life.
- Track your progress. Keep a food journal to note what you eat and how you feel. This might allow you to identify trigger foods and patterns in your symptoms.
- Find a support system. Talk to your doctor, a qualified nutritionist, or a support group for people with acid reflux. Having somebody to chat with can help you keep motivated and on track.

How to handle setbacks

Everyone experiences obstacles from time to time. If you experience a setback, don't give up. Just pick yourself up and start again. Here are a few tips for handling setbacks:

- Don't beat yourself up. Everyone makes errors. It is vital to forgive oneself and move on.
- Identify what caused the setback. Once you know what caused the setback, you may start to design tactics for preventing it in the future.
- Get back on track as quickly as possible. Don't let a setback disrupt your development. Just pick yourself up and start over as quickly as possible.

Finding support

Having a support system can be useful when following the acid reflux diet. There are a variety of venues where you can find support.

- Your doctor or registered dietician Your doctor or registered dietitian can give you information about the acid reflux diet and help you build a plan that is ideal for you.

- Support groups. There are a variety of support groups for those with acid reflux. These groups might offer you a secure area to share your experiences and learn from others.
- Online communities. There are also a lot of online communities for people with acid reflux. These communities can be a terrific way to connect with people who are going through the same thing.

Following the acid reflux diet for the long run can be tough, but it is worth it to manage your symptoms and enhance your general health. By following the guidelines above, you can boost your chances of long-term success.

CHAPTER 7

ACID RELUX DIET RECIPE FOR THE WHOLE FAMILY

Breakfast Recipes

- Oatmeal with berries and nuts: This is a classic breakfast that is both nutritious and delicious. Oatmeal is a good source of fiber, which can help alleviate acid reflux symptoms. Berries and nuts are also wonderful sources of antioxidants and other minerals.
- Yogurt with fruit and granola: Yogurt is another fantastic source of protein and fiber. It is also a good source of probiotics, which can help enhance intestinal health. Fruit and granola are good sources of vitamins and minerals.
- Smoothies made with fruits, veggies, and yogurt: Smoothies are a terrific way to obtain a quick and nutritious breakfast. Be cautious when using fruits and vegetables that are low in acid. You may also add yogurt to your smoothie for extra protein and probiotics.

Lunch Recipes

- Salad with grilled chicken or fish: Salads are a terrific way to receive a range of nutrients in one meal. Be cautious when using low-acid dressings and toppings. Grilled chicken or fish is a fantastic source of protein.
- Soup and sandwich: Soup is an excellent method to warm up on a cold day. Be cautious when choosing a soup that is low in fat and acid. You can also enjoy a sandwich on whole-wheat bread with lean protein and low-fat cheese.
- Leftovers from dinner: Leftovers can be a quick and easy lunch alternative. Just be sure to reheat them thoroughly.

Dinner Recipes

- Grilled salmon with roasted vegetables: Salmon is a high source of omega-3 fatty acids, which can help reduce inflammation. Roasted veggies are a good source of vitamins and minerals.
- Chicken stir-fry with brown rice: Stir-fries are a quick and easy way to make a healthy supper. Be sure to use low-acid sauces and oils. Brown rice is a good source of fiber.
- Pasta with tomato sauce and meatballs: Pasta is a staple cuisine for many families. Just be sure to use a low-acid tomato sauce and lean meatballs.

These are just a few examples of acid reflux diet recipes for the whole family.

Here are some additional recommendations for cooking acid-reflux diet-friendly meals:

- Use low-acid substances. This includes fruits, vegetables, meats, and dairy items.
- Avoid processed meals. Processed foods are generally heavy in harmful fats, sugar, and acid.
- Cook at home as often as possible. This gives you more control over the ingredients in your diet.
- Eat small, frequent meals. This can help minimize acid production and prevent stomach acid from backing up into your esophagus.

By following these recommendations, you may cook healthful and delicious meals that everyone will love, including those with acid reflux.

CHAPTER 8

ACID RELUX DIET MEAL PLANS FOR DIFFERENT LIFESTYLE

Meal Plan for Busy Professionals

Here is a typical meal plan for busy professionals on the acid reflux diet:

Breakfast:

- Oatmeal with berries and nuts
- Smoothie composed of fruits, veggies, and yogurt
- Hard-boiled eggs with whole-wheat bread and avocado

Lunch:

Salad with grilled chicken or fish
Soup and sandwich on whole-wheat bread with lean protein and low-fat cheese
Leftovers from dinner

Dinner:

- Grilled salmon with roasted veggies
- Chicken stir-fry with brown rice
- Pasta with tomato sauce and meatballs

Snacks:

- Fruits and vegetables
- Yogurt Nuts

Meal Plan for Families

Here is a typical meal plan for families on the acid reflux diet:

Breakfast:

- Oatmeal with berries and nuts
- Yogurt with fruit and granola
- Whole-wheat waffles with peanut butter and banana

Lunch:

- Grilled chicken salad sandwiches on whole-wheat bread
- Soup and salad
- Leftovers from supper

Dinner:

- Spaghetti with low-acid tomato sauce and meatballs
- Chicken stir-fry with brown rice
- Salmon with roasted veggies

Snacks:

- Fruits and vegetables
- Yogurt Hard-boiled eggs
- Meal Plan for Students

Here is a sample meal plan for students on the acid reflux diet:

Breakfast:

- Oatmeal with berries and nuts
- Yogurt with fruit and granola
- Whole-wheat bread with avocado

Lunch:

- Salad with grilled chicken or fish
- Soup and sandwich on whole-wheat bread with lean protein and low-fat cheese
- Leftovers from dinner

Dinner:

- Pasta with low-acid tomato sauce and meatballs
- Chicken stir-fry with brown rice
- Salmon with roasted veggies

Snacks:

- Fruits and vegetables
- Yogurt
- Hard-boiled eggs

These are just a few samples of meal plans for diverse lifestyles on the acid reflux diet.

Here are some extra recommendations for following the acid reflux diet on the go:

- Cook in quantity on the weekends. This will save you time during the week.
- Pack your meals and snacks ahead of time. This can enable you to avoid making bad decisions when you are hungry and on the road.
- Choose healthful convenience foods. There are a lot of healthy convenience foods available, such as pre-cut fruits and vegetables, whole-wheat bread, and low-fat dairy products.
- Don't be afraid to ask for accommodations. If you are eating out, ask your

server for changes, such as no butter or cheese on your food.

By following these suggestions, you may follow the acid reflux diet and control your symptoms, even if you have a hectic lifestyle.

SUMMARY

The acid reflux diet is a technique to control acid reflux symptoms by avoiding trigger meals and consuming foods that are low in acid. In addition to the food, there are a variety of lifestyle modifications that can help to lessen acid reflux symptoms, such as stopping smoking, lowering weight, managing stress, avoiding eating late at night, and elevating the head of your bed at night.

If you experience acid reflux, it is vital to talk to your doctor or registered dietitian to build a strategy that is ideal for you. They can help you to identify your trigger foods, design a meal plan, and provide support while you make adjustments to your diet and lifestyle.

Here are some extra tips for following the acid reflux diet and controlling acid reflux symptoms:

- Eat modest, frequent meals throughout the day. This will assist to lower the quantity of acid in your stomach at any one time.
- Avoid lying down within three hours of eating. This will assist to prevent stomach acid from backing up into your esophagus.
- Drink plenty of water throughout the day. Water can assist to dilute stomach acid and make it less likely to irritate your esophagus.
- Avoid caffeine and alcohol. Caffeine and alcohol can relax the lower esophageal sphincter (LES), which can allow stomach acid to back up into your esophagus.
- Identify and avoid your trigger foods. Common trigger foods include fatty foods, spicy foods, citrus fruits, tomatoes, chocolate, coffee, and tea.
- Manage stress. Stress might trigger acid reflux symptoms. Find healthy strategies to manage stress, such as exercise, relaxation techniques, and spending time with loved ones.

Following the acid reflux diet and adopting lifestyle adjustments will assist you to control your acid reflux symptoms and improving your quality of life.